Restless Legs Syndrome

All You Need To Know

Disclaimer

This content serves to provide general information about the disease and aims to empower you to seek prompt medical assistance if necessary to prevent complications. It's essential to stress that this information is not a substitute for consulting a qualified physician. The field of medical science is continually evolving, and due to the dynamic nature of medical knowledge, we recommend seeking expert advice if you encounter any inconsistencies or intend to take action based on the information in this content. Never disregard professional medical guidance or delay treatment based on something you've read online, including this material, or from any other online source. Always remember that the internet cannot cure you; rather, healing comes through the guidance of medical professionals and the providence of God.

Table of Contents

Introduction

The neurological disorder known as Restless Legs Syndrome (RLS), which is typified by an overwhelming desire to move the legs, is a mysterious and puzzling ailment that has baffled medical experts as well as those who suffer from it. Even though RLS is the most common name for this ailment, "Willis-Ekbom disease" is another name for it. The historical contributions of two medical professionals—English physician Sir Thomas Willis from the 17th century and Swedish neurologist Karl-Axel Ekbom from the 20th century—are responsible for the introduction of this alternate word.

Why is Restless Legs Syndrome (RLS) also called Willis-Ekbom Disease?

Among the first to describe the strange sensations and leg movements linked to RLS was Sir Thomas Willis. He painstakingly recorded the experiences of people who described their legs as "restless" and stated an overwhelming desire to move them in order to relieve discomfort in his 1672 work "De Anima Brutorum." Future research on this condition was made possible by his astute observations.

Karl-Axel Ekbom, on the other hand, made important advances in the middle of the 20th century by offering a more thorough clinical description of the illness. Our knowledge of RLS was expanded by Ekbom's study, which was also essential in helping to differentiate it from other neurological disorders.

To celebrate the landmark work of Sir Thomas Willis and Karl-Axel Ekbom, RLS was given the alternate term "Willis-Ekbom disease" in appreciation of their substantial contributions to the study of this ailment. The title Willis-Ekbom disease honors the historical history and ongoing contributions of these two significant people in the area of neurology, even though RLS is still the more widely used word.

Section 1

Prevalence and Impact of RLS

Millions of individuals throughout the world suffer from the ailment known as restless legs syndrome. Despite its seemingly innocent name, this neurological condition can have a major influence on the everyday lives of those who are affected. Unexpectedly, RLS is more widespread than one might think, and its effects can be severe.

In the general population, the prevalence of restless legs syndrome (RLS) varies between 5 and 15%. The frequency of RLS in various age groups and communities has been documented in a number of studies and surveys. People with this illness might come from a variety of cultures, origins, and geographical locations. It affects people of all ages equally, therefore it should worry both young and old. RLS is an equal-opportunity condition that affects people of all sexes.

One cannot overestimate the influence of RLS on day-to-day living. The constant need to move one's legs and the pain that goes along with it can cause problems in many areas of life, including employment, social interactions, sleep, and general wellbeing. Living with this neurological condition comes with its own set of obstacles.

Section 2

Symptoms of RLS

An accurate diagnosis depends on a thorough grasp of the symptoms, which are the primary indicators of the illness. Here are a few of the main symptoms:

- **Irresistible Urge to Move the Legs:** The incessant and almost uncontrollable need to move the legs is the fundamental cause of RLS. The hallmark of the illness is this urge, which usually appears when the patient is at rest, as when they are sitting or lying down. It's usually described as a very painful and strong feeling that forces people to move their legs in an attempt to find relief.

- **Sensations in the Legs:** Many strange feelings in the legs are another feature of RLS. Although it might be difficult to describe these feelings, words like "creeping," "crawling," "itching," and "tingling" are commonly used. They add to the pain and agitation that people with RLS go through.

Effects and Experiences of Symptoms

It's critical to keep in mind that RLS symptoms can vary greatly in subjective experience, and that not everyone feels the same way or to the same extent. The insatiable need to move the legs in order to alleviate these sensations, however, is a defining feature of RLS. This movement compulsivity is a hallmark of RLS and frequently distinguishes it from other disorders

- **Sensations of Crawling or Creeping:** People with RLS frequently talk about feeling as though there are insects crawling on or just under their skin. This feeling can be quite disturbing and uncomfortable.

- **Tingling or Electric Sensations:** A few RLS sufferers describe their tingling sensations as being similar to an electric current passing through their legs. These feelings may be unpleasant and harsh.

- **Itching:** One of the most prevalent complaints from people with RLS is itching in the legs. Even in situations where there isn't any obvious skin irritation, this itching can be severe and enduring.

- **Aching or Throbbing Pain:** A deep, achy, or throbbing ache that sometimes affects patients with RLS is described as occurring in their legs. The severity and intermittent nature of this discomfort are both possible.

- **Restlessness:** The term "restless" in Restless Leg Syndrome is quite fitting. Individuals often experience a constant, nagging discomfort in their legs, making it challenging to sit or lie still, especially in the evening and at night.

When a person is at rest, such as when sitting or lying down, these RLS feelings are usually the most noticeable, and they usually get worse in the evening or at night. The pain may be so severe that it keeps you from falling asleep, which can result in persistent sleep disorders including insomnia.

Section 3

Causes Of RLS

Primary Causes

The neurological disorder known as restless legs syndrome (RLS) has numerous, intricate causes. Although the specific cause of RLS is not fully understood, research has identified a number of potential risk factors. It's crucial to remember that any one of the following causes may contribute to RLS:

- **Genetics:** Since RLS has a significant hereditary component, it may run in families. Certain gene variations that have been identified as enhancing vulnerability to RLS include MEIS1, BTBD9, and MAP2K5/SKOR1. It is crucial to comprehend the impact that genetics plays in RLS since it can increase awareness of risk and encourage early identification and treatment for those who have a family history of the disorder.

- **Dopamine Imbalance:** RLS has been linked to changes in the brain's dopamine levels, a neurotransmitter. Since dopamine is a key neurotransmitter in controlling muscle activity, abnormalities in this neurotransmitter may play a role in the emergence of RLS symptoms.

- **Iron Deficiency:** One frequent secondary cause of RLS is an iron deficit. Inadequate iron levels in the body can interfere with dopamine generation and function. Iron deficiency must be identified and treated when it occurs since iron therapy can frequently reduce or eliminate RLS symptoms.

- **Pregnancy:** RLS may develop or worsen while a woman is pregnant. Pregnant women may experience hormonal fluctuations that impact the development of RLS symptoms, such as increased estrogen levels. Pregnant women and healthcare professionals should be aware of this information since treating RLS during pregnancy may call for a different strategy.

Secondary Causes of RLS

Numerous secondary disorders or circumstances can potentially cause or worsen Restless Legs Syndrome. It is essential to comprehend these secondary reasons in order to manage effectively:

- **Medication-Induced RLS:** A number of pharmaceuticals, such as antipsychotics, antiemetic medications, and some antidepressants, have been connected to the onset of RLS symptoms in certain people. It's crucial to be aware of the possibility of medication-induced RLS because these symptoms are frequently relieved by modifying or stopping prescriptions.

- **Chronic Illnesses:** Peripheral neuropathy, diabetes, and renal disease are examples of chronic illnesses that can exacerbate RLS. Controlling these underlying illnesses is necessary to properly control the symptoms of RLS.

- **Lifestyle and Environmental Factors:** RLS symptoms can be exacerbated by lifestyle choices such as smoking, sleep deprivation, and excessive alcohol or caffeine usage. For those with RLS, addressing these variables can greatly enhance their quality of life.

Section 4

Diagnosis of Restless Legs Syndrome (RLS)

Making the diagnosis of restless legs syndrome is essential to offering the right kind of assistance and care. A thorough assessment consists of the following:

- **Clinical Assessment:** The diagnosis is mostly based on a clinical evaluation. Medical professionals obtain a thorough medical history, which includes details regarding the type and timing of RLS symptoms.

- **Physical Examination:** To rule out other possible reasons of leg discomfort, such as neuropathy or circulation problems, a physical examination is performed.

- **The International Restless Legs Scale (IRLS):** This approved measure aids in determining the degree of RLS symptoms and how they affect a person's day-to-day activities.

- **Polysomnography:** To evaluate sleep patterns and rule out other sleep disorders, such as periodic limb movement disorder, a polysomnography sleep study may be performed in certain circumstances.

- **Laboratory Tests:** Iron deficiency can be a major contributing factor to RLS, hence blood tests may be conducted to evaluate iron levels.

- **Differential Diagnosis:** To differentiate RLS from illnesses that resemble its symptoms, like periodic limb movement disorder and nocturnal leg cramps, differential diagnosis is essential.

To give them the best possible care and management techniques, a precise diagnosis of RLS is necessary. This will help them take back control of their lives and lessen the effects of the illness. The heart and brain are two other areas where restless leg syndrome may have an impact. For this reason, if you encounter the symptoms, you must see a doctor right away.

Differential Diagnosis of RLS

In order to correctly diagnose Restless Legs Syndrome (RLS), differential diagnosis is essential since it makes sure that other illnesses that may cause similar symptoms are ruled out. This is a synopsis of this feature:

- **RLS vs. Nocturnal Leg Cramps:** RLS symptoms can occasionally be mistaken for nocturnal leg cramps. Leg cramps, on the other hand, are usually not the same as the typical RLS feelings; instead, they are usually sudden, strong, and painful muscle spasms.

- **RLS vs. Periodic Limb Movement Disorder (PLMD):**Another movement disorder associated with sleep, PLMD is typified by involuntary, repetitive leg motions while you sleep. Even though PLMD and RLS can co-occur, they are two different illnesses. While PLMD comprises limb movements during sleep without the conscious need to move, RLS predominantly involves a need to move the legs while awake.

Section 5

Treatment and Management

Improving the quality of life for individuals afflicted with RLS requires effective care of the condition. This section examines several forms of treatment:

Non-Medical Approaches

Non-medical strategies are often the first line of treatment for RLS, and they include:

- **Lifestyle Modifications:** This may entail abstaining from or consuming less alcohol and caffeine, as these substances might aggravate symptoms. It's also critical to keep a regular sleep routine and furnish a cozy sleeping space.

- **Exercise:** Walking and other moderate-intensity exercises are examples of regular physical activity that might help reduce RLS symptoms by enhancing circulation and general wellbeing. But be careful not to go overboard.

- **Sleep Hygiene:** Making a sleep-friendly environment, cutting back on screen time before bed, and making sure the bedroom is quiet, cold, and dark are all parts of excellent sleep hygiene.

- **Iron Supplementation:** To treat this underlying reason, iron supplements may be suggested for people who are iron deficient.

The importance of these non-medical strategies cannot be overstated, as they can significantly reduce the impact of RLS on daily life.

Medical Approaches

When Non-Medical Approaches are insufficient, or symptoms are severe, healthcare providers may prescribe medications. Common medications for RLS include:

- **Dopaminergic Agents:** RLS symptoms may be lessened by drugs that alter dopamine levels in the brain, such as ropinirole and pramipexole.

- **Opioids:** Opioids may be administered in situations of severe RLS, but because of the possibility of side effects and dependence, these are usually only used as a last resort.

- **Anticonvulsants:** It has been discovered that some anticonvulsant drugs, such as gabapentin, are useful in treating RLS symptoms.

Since everyone reacts to drugs differently, customized treatment strategies are essential. Carefully weighing the advantages, disadvantages, and side effects is necessary.

Alternative and Complementary Medicine

Alternative and Complementary Medicine can complement conventional treatments and may include:

- **Acupuncture:** Tiny needles are inserted into particular body spots during the age-old practice of acupuncture in order to relieve symptoms. Acupuncture sessions can provide relief for some people suffering from RLS.

- **Massage:** A light leg massage might enhance relaxation and offer momentary relief from RLS symptoms

- **Cognitive-Behavioral Therapy (CBT):** People with RLS may find it difficult to handle the psychological and emotional effects of their condition, such as worry and sleep difficulties. CBT approaches can help.

These treatments should be customized to each patient's needs and preferences and are best undertaken under the supervision of licensed professionals.

But there are also a lot of misconceptions regarding non-traditional approaches to treating restless legs syndrome. Any home remedies should be thoroughly researched before being chosen over therapies based on scientific evidence.

To sum up, treating RLS is a complex process that requires differential diagnosis to identify it from other illnesses that are similar.

The cornerstone of treatment is non-pharmacological methods like exercise, sleep hygiene, and lifestyle changes. When required, pharmaceutical interventions and complementary therapies can alleviate symptoms and enhance the standard of living for people with RLS. Tailored therapy regimens are necessary, considering the distinct requirements and reactions of every patient.

Section 6

RLS Pain and Medication-Induced RLS

This section explores the pain that some people with restless legs syndrome (RLS) experience, as well as how certain drugs may cause or exacerbate RLS symptoms.

Pain in Restless Legs Syndrome

The symptoms of restless legs syndrome usually include painful sensations and an overwhelming need to move the legs. But another important aspect of the RLS experience might also involve discomfort. RLS-related pain can range in intensity from little discomfort to excruciating distress.

- **Mild Discomfort:** Many RLS sufferers characterize the pain as a persistent annoyance that is akin to an itching or annoying feeling. Although it's normally not severe, it can be ongoing, which makes it challenging to unwind and locate comfort.

- **Aching and Throbbing:** Some people may experience a greater degree of pain, causing their legs to ache and throb. This can be quite upsetting for people, especially at night when they're attempting to fall asleep.

- **Burning and Pricking:** RLS pain can have a burning or prickling feeling in more extreme situations. This kind of pain can be depressing and difficult to control.

Healthcare professionals and those who have RLS must both comprehend the type of pain that the disorder causes. It makes it possible to diagnose conditions with greater accuracy and to create specialized management plans that reduce suffering and enhance quality of life.

Medication-Induced RLS

RLS symptoms have been related to the onset or exacerbation of certain drugs. The main topic of this subsection is the ways in which certain drugs, such as antipsychotics, antiemetic medications, and antidepressants, can cause or worsen RLS.

- **Antipsychotics:** There has been evidence linking certain antipsychotic drugs, particularly those from the earlier generation, to RLS symptoms. For those in need of antipsychotic therapy for illnesses such as bipolar disorder or schizophrenia, this can pose a challenging situation because controlling RLS symptoms becomes essential to their general health.

- **Anti-Nausea Drugs:** RLS symptoms can be exacerbated by several anti-nausea medications, especially those that impact the dopaminergic system. These drugs are frequently administered for ailments like chemotherapy- or pregnancy-related nausea.

- **Antidepressants:** It has been observed that certain antidepressants, particularly selective serotonin reuptake inhibitors (SSRIs), might worsen or even cause RLS symptoms. For those who are suffering from both depression and RLS, this poses a problem because they need to carefully weigh their therapy alternatives.

Making well-informed treatment decisions requires being able to recognize medication-induced RLS. In these situations, medical professionals might have to look at different drugs or methods of treatment to take care of the underlying issue while reducing the effect on RLS symptoms.

Section 7

Coping Mechanisms and Assistance

This section describes coping mechanisms and emphasizes the psychological and emotional elements of having RLS. It also highlights how crucial it is to establish support systems.

Coping with RLS

Addressing the emotional and psychological effects that RLS may have on people is part of coping with the illness. The chronic nature of RLS can cause annoyance, worry, and even melancholy. It can also interfere with sleep and daily activities.

- **Emotional Impact:** RLS can cause emotional exhaustion. Its difficulties might cause people to feel irritated, nervous, and even alone. Coping mechanisms that target these feelings will improve people's general state of wellbeing.

- **Psychological Impact:** Fatigue and cognitive difficulties can be brought on by RLS-induced sleep disruptions. Coping strategies must take into account the psychological effects, emphasizing resilience and mental health.

- **Daily Life:** Individuals can control the impact of RLS on their everyday routines by using practical coping strategies. This covers methods for managing sleep, interacting with people, and working.

Support Networks

Getting help is a vital part of managing RLS. The significance of obtaining support from medical professionals, support groups, and internet communities is emphasized in this part.

- **Healthcare Providers:** Neurologists and sleep specialists are among the medical professionals that can offer advice, diagnosis, and treatment choices. Building a reliable healthcare team is necessary for efficient administration.

- **Support Groups:** Participating in RLS support groups can be quite helpful. By giving people a forum to discuss their experiences, coping mechanisms, and insights, these organizations promote understanding and a feeling of community.

- **Online Communities:** People can interact with others, pose questions, and obtain important data and resources through online RLS forums and communities.

Section 8

The Prospects for RLS Studies

Research on RLS could lead to significant progress in our knowledge of and ability to treat the disorder in the future. The goal of this research is to learn more about the causes of RLS, possible remedies, and the creation of more potent medications. The field of RLS research is constantly changing, with ongoing studies, genetics-related inquiries, and a better comprehension of the underlying mechanisms of RLS all playing important roles. It's critical to monitor these changes since they could influence how RLS is diagnosed and treated in the future. Research directions consist of:

- **Genetics and Biomarkers:** Important new information on the genesis of RLS may come from ongoing studies on the genetic components linked to the disorder. Finding biomarkers may improve diagnosis and result in more specialized care.

- **Neurological Mechanisms:** The discovery of novel therapeutics for RLS requires a clearer knowledge of the brain mechanisms underlying the condition. Studies look at the functions of neurotransmitters, especially dopamine, and how symptoms of RLS are related to them.

- **Pharmacological Innovations:** A sizable portion of RLS research focuses on examining novel drugs and therapeutic modalities. Researchers are looking at cutting-edge medications and treatments that may offer more effective symptom relief.

- **Non-Pharmacological Interventions:** Additionally, studies are examining the effectiveness of non-pharmacological treatments such acupuncture, lifestyle changes, and cognitive-behavioral therapy (CBT). These methods are thought to be viable complimentary techniques for managing RLS.

Section 9
Conclusion

To sum up, restless legs syndrome, or RLS, is a complicated neurological disorder that affects people differently. It's critical for medical professionals and RLS patients alike to comprehend RLS pain and medication-induced RLS. Pain can range from moderate discomfort to more severe misery in RLS patients, and certain drugs can cause or worsen RLS symptoms, creating special difficulties.

Finding workable coping mechanisms for everyday life and attending to the emotional and psychological effects of RLS are key components of coping with the illness. Effective RLS management is greatly aided by support networks, which include medical professionals, support groups, and online communities.

With studies examining genetics, neurological causes, novel pharmaceuticals, and non-pharmacological therapies underway, the future of RLS research seems bright. These developments could lead to better RLS diagnosis and therapy, which would ultimately enhance the condition's impact on sufferers' quality of life.

Section 10

FAQs On Restless Legs Syndrome (RLS)

1. Does Diabetes affect RLS?

Diabetes's affects on blood vessel and nerve function can affect RLS. Elevated blood glucose levels could worsen the symptoms of RLS. Improved RLS control can result from diabetes management, including food, exercise, and medication.

2. Is there a link between high cholesterol and RLS?

While high cholesterol doesn't directly cause RLS, it can worsen symptoms. Cholesterol plaques in blood vessels may affect circulation, potentially intensifying RLS discomfort. Maintaining a healthy diet, exercising, and managing cholesterol levels can support RLS management.

3. How does the liver impact RLS?

Liver conditions, like iron overload or cirrhosis, can lead to RLS due to their effects on iron regulation. Treating liver issues and monitoring iron levels is essential in managing RLS symptoms. Collaborating with a healthcare provider is crucial for comprehensive care.

4. Can Kidney problems worsen RLS?

Kidney problems can disrupt iron balance in the body, potentially worsening RLS. Individuals with kidney issues should work closely with healthcare providers to manage their kidney health and monitor iron levels. Addressing these factors may help alleviate RLS symptoms.

5. Does RLS affect bone health?

RLS itself doesn't directly affect bone health, but the sleep disturbances it causes can lead to chronic fatigue. Prolonged fatigue may indirectly impact bone health over time. Maintaining a balanced diet, regular exercise, and good sleep hygiene can help mitigate these effects and support overall well-being.

6. What's the connection between RLS and the heart?

RLS has been associated with an increased risk of cardiovascular issues, possibly due to its impact on sleep quality and patterns. Managing RLS and addressing sleep disturbances is important for supporting heart health. Lifestyle modifications and collaborating with healthcare providers are key components of a heart-healthy approach for individuals with RLS.

www.ingramcontent.com/pod-product-compliance
Lightning Source LLC
Chambersburg PA
CBHW070754260726
48660CB00007B/3113